RENAL DIET COOKBOOK FOR BEGINNERS

Delicious Recipes to Control Kidney Disease and Live Healthier Avoiding Dialysis.

(Second Edition)

Diamond DeJesus

TABLE OF CONTENTS

WHAT IS RENAL DIET?

This diet can help decrease the rate of kidney damage. The diet may change over time as the health condition changes. You may also need to make other dietary changes if you have other health problems, such as diabetes. Dietary therapy is one of the important treatments for kidney disease. A correct and reasonable diet can reduce water and electrolyte disorders, reduce proteinuria, relieve clinical symptoms, and stop the progression of renal disease.

How Does It Work?

A proper diet is necessary for controlling the amount of toxic waste in the bloodstream. When toxic waste piles up in the system along with increased fluid, chronic inflammation occurs, and we will be more prone to have cardiovascular, bone, metabolic, or other health issues.

Since your kidneys can't fully get rid of waste on their own, which comes from food and drinks, probably the only natural way to help our system is through this diet.

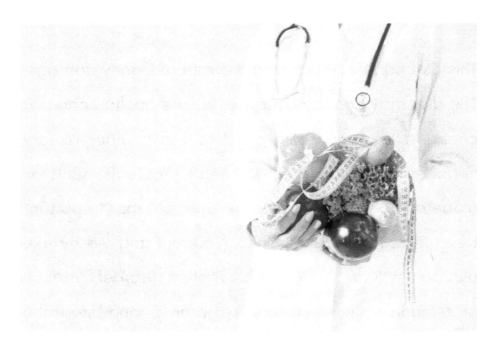

A renal diet is especially useful during the first stages of kidney dysfunction and leads to the following benefits:

☐   Prevents excess fluid and waste build-up.

☐   Prevents the progression of renal dysfunction stages.

☐   Decreases the likelihood of developing other chronic health problems, e.g., heart disorders

☐ Has a mild antioxidant function in the body, which keeps inflammation and inflammatory responses under control.

The above-mentioned benefits are noticeable once the patient follows the diet for at least a month and then continuing it for longer periods to avoid the stage where dialysis is needed. The strictness of the diet depends on the current stage of renal/kidney disease, if, for example, you are in the 3rd or 4th stage, you should follow a stricter diet and be attentive to the food, which is allowed or prohibited.

Benefits

Doctors and dietitians have developed a diet that helps their patients with compromised kidney function cut down the amount of waste that their body produces that their kidneys can't filter out. A renal diet is lower in sodium, phosphorus, and protein than a typical diet. Every person's body is different, which means that what works for one person will not work for another. Some people have to cut their levels of potassium and calcium as well.

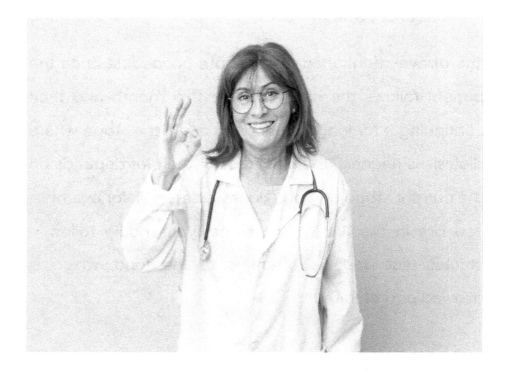

A renal diet must be tailored to meet the individual needs and toxin levels of the patient. Keeping a food journal may become necessary and is highly recommended. Sometimes it can be hard to keep track of all of the foods and their amounts; a journal can make keeping track a lot less intimidating. A physical notebook or even a cell phone application can be used for this.

Sodium (mg)

Sodium and table salt are two different components. Table salt is comprised of sodium and chloride. However, sodium by itself is a mineral that is naturally occurring in most of the foods that we eat. That is the reason why processed foods are not recommended for someone with kidney problems or in a renal diet due to the added salt that is put into them.

Sodium is one of three major electrolytes that help control the fluids going in and out of the cells and tissue in the body. Sodium is responsible for helping control blood pressure and volume, muscle contraction and nerve functions, regulating the acid and base balance of the blood, and balancing the elimination and retention of fluid in the body.

Renal patients are required to monitor their sodium intake because when the kidney's functions become compromised, it is harder for their body to eliminate the fluids and the sodium that is in excess in the body.

It has side effects that include:

- Increased thirst
- Edema
- High blood pressure
- Shortness of breath from fluid being retained in the lungs
- Heart failure from an overworked and weak heart that has had to work harder due to the body making it work harder.

Limiting sodium can be easier than you think. Since sodium content is always listed on food labels, it is important to get into the habit of checking not only sodium content but the single serving size as well. As a rule of thumb, fresh is better. Packaged foods typically have added salt, so stick with things that have no salt added to them.

Start comparing the items you use. If it is a spice, steer clear of something with "salt" in the title. When you are cooking in your home, do not add extra salt to your food under any circumstance. Too much sodium can make chronic kidney disease progress much faster.

Potassium (mg)

Potassium is another of the three major electrolytes in the body. It is a naturally occurring mineral found in many foods and in our own bodies. Potassium helps keep our hearts beating regularly and our muscles working correctly. The kidneys have a duty when regulating the amount of potassium in the body.

These organs, when healthy, know just how much potassium your body needs. Excess potassium is cleansed from the body through the body's urine output. When you have chronic kidney disease, this naturally occurring regulation in the body becomes compromised.

Hyperkalemia, come with the following symptoms:

☐ Weakness in the muscles

☐ Irregular heartbeat

- A pulse that is slower than normal

- Heart attack/Stroke

- Death Learning how to limit potassium, just like sodium, is an important part of your renal diet.

Foods like bananas, fish, spinach, avocados, and potatoes are high in potassium and are foods to avoid. Cut down on your milk and dairy consumption to eight ounces per day. Make sure to read the labels and adhere to the single serving size of the foods you are eating.

Phosphorus (mg)

Phosphorus is a mineral that aids the bones and the muscles in the body. When food is ingested, the small intestines absorb the amount of phosphorus needed for the bones, but the kidneys are in charge of removing the extra phosphorus. When the kidneys can't expel the extra phosphorus, it builds up in the blood and pulls calcium from the bones, making them weak. High amounts of phosphorus can also cause calcium deposits to build up in the heart, lungs, eyes, and blood vessels.

Keeping phosphorus levels low, just like sodium and potassium, is important in a renal diet. Stop eating foods that are rich in phosphorus like soda, cheese, meat, milk, and seeds. It may be necessary to discuss using phosphate binders with your doctor to keep your levels under control. Make sure to avoid foods with added phosphorus. These will be labeled with "PHOS" on the label.

Protein (g)

Protein levels can be a tricky thing to keep equaled out if you have chronic kidney disease. Different stages of CKD tolerate protein levels differently and depending on which stage of CKD you are experiencing your diet will reflect a different level of proteins allowed. Proteins are important to the body, so you can't eliminate them from your diet. You can be aware of your intake and what your body can tolerate and what it can't.

Fluid

It is important for fluid intake to be strictly monitored due to the probability of the fluid being retained in the body. When a person is on dialysis, their urine output is decreased, so extra fluid can cause unnecessary strain on the body. Fluid intake levels will be calculated by a nutritionist or doctor on a personal basis. Never drink more than what the doctor tells you is okay, and do not forget to consider solids that turn to liquid at room temperature or used in cooking.

JUICE, SMOOTHIE & DRINK RECIPES

Blackberry Sage Water

Prep time: 10 min | Cooking time: 0 min | Servings: 10

NUTRITION PER SERVING:

Calories 24 | Total Fat 0.3g | Saturated Fat 0.1g | Cholesterol 0mg | Sodium 1mg | Carbohydrate 2.9g | Dietary Fiber 1.6g | Sugars 1.9g | Protein 0.4g | Calcium 28mg | Phosphorous 13mg | Potassium 48mg.

Ingredients

15 medium fresh sage leaves

2 tsp. stevia

1 cup boiling water

6 oz. fresh blackberries.

Directions

1. Add the sage leaves, stevia, blackberries, and water to a blender jug.

1. Blend well, then strain and refrigerate to chill.

2. Serve.

Watermelon Mint Drink

Prep time: 5 min | Cooking time: 0 min | Servings: 2

NUTRITION PER SERVING:

Calories 148 | Total Fat 0.6g | Saturated Fat 0.3g | Cholesterol 0mg | Sodium 11mg | Carbohydrate 38g | Dietary Fiber 2g | Sugars 28.7g | Protein 2.9g | Calcium 41mg | Phosphorous 24mg | Potassium 559mg.

Ingredients

6 cups seedless watermelon, cubed

2 limes juice

1 cup water.

Directions

1. First, begin by putting everything into a blender jug.

2. Pulse it for 30 seconds until well blended.

3. Serve chilled.

Caramel Latte

Prep time: 10 min | Cooking time: 0 min | Servings: 1

NUTRITION PER SERVING:

Calories 217 | Total Fat 4.3g | Saturated Fat 2.8g | Cholesterol 15mg | Sodium 166mg | Carbohydrate 32.8g | Dietary Fiber 0.2g | Sugars 16.4g | Protein 4.6g | Calcium 168mg | Phosphorous 41mg | Potassium 217mg.

Ingredients

½ cup almond milk

1 tbsp. brown Swerve

1 tbsp. caramel topping

1 tbsp. caramel sauce

¼ tsp. vanilla extract

1 cup coffee.

Directions

1. Heat the milk in a 1-quart saucepan over moderate heat and add the Swerve, vanilla extract, and coffee.

2. Cook this latte up to a boil then pour into the serving mug.

3. Top it with caramel and sauce.

4. Enjoy.

Peach Raspberry Smoothie

Prep time: 10 min | Cooking time: 0 min | Servings: 3

NUTRITION PER SERVING:

Calories 129 | Total Fat 3.2g | Sodium 53mg | Carbohydrate 23g | Protein 6.3g | Phosphorous 72mg | Potassium 261mg.

Ingredients

1 cup frozen raspberries

1 medium peach, pit removed, sliced

½ cup tofu

1 tbsp. honey (or stevia)

1 cup unfortified almond milk.

Directions

1. Put all ingredients into a blender jug.

2. Mix until smooth.

Pina Colada Smoothie

Prep time: 10 min | Cooking time: 0 min | Servings: 2

NUTRITION PER SERVING:

Calories: 189g | Protein: 13.4g | Carbohydrates: 32g | Fibre: 3g | Total Fat: 5g | Sodium: 5mg | Phosphorus: 121mg | Potassium: 349 mg.

Ingredients

1 cup fresh pineapple

1 cup (8 oz) tofu, firm

½ cup pineapple juice, unsweetened

1 tsp. Stevia

1 pinch of red pepper flakes.

Directions

1. First, begin by putting everything into a blender jug.

2. Pulse it for 30 seconds until well blended.

3. Serve chilled.

Pineapple Sorbet Smoothie

Prep time: 10 min | Cooking time: 0 min | Servings: 1

NUTRITION PER SERVING:

Calories 180 | Total Fat 1g | Saturated Fat 0.5g | Cholesterol 40mg | Sodium 86mg | Carbohydrate 30.5g | Dietary Fiber 0g | Sugars 28g | Protein 13g | Calcium 9mg | Phosphorous 164mg | Potassium 111mg.

Ingredients

¾ cup pineapple sorbet

1 scoop protein powder

½ cup water

2 ice cubes, optional.

Directions

1. First, begin by putting everything into a blender jug.

1. Pulse it for 30 seconds until well blended.

2. Serve chilled.

Lemon Apple Honey Smoothie

Prep time: 10 min | Cooking time: 0 min | Servings: 4

NUTRITION PER SERVING:

Calories 170 | Fat 1g | Sodium 37mg | Carbohydrates 38g | Dietary Fiber 2g | | Protein 2g | Phosphorous 59mg | Potassium 327mg.

Ingredients

¼ cup lemon juice

½ cup apple juice

1 apple, peeled and cored

1 banana

2-3 tsp. honey

1 cup low-fat vanilla yogurt, frozen.

Directions

1. Combine all ingredients in a blender and mix until smooth.

2. Serve immediately.

BEST
BREAKFAST
RECIPES

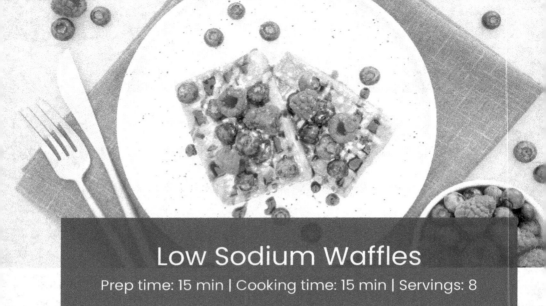

Low Sodium Waffles

Prep time: 15 min | Cooking time: 15 min | Servings: 8

NUTRITION PER SERVING:

Calories: 173 | Fat: 5.2g | Sodium: 31.2mg | Carbs: 26g | Protein: 5g | Potassium 178mg | Phosphorus 82mg.

Ingredients

1¾ cups all-purpose flour

2 tbsp. stevia

2 tbsp. sodium-free baking powder

2 eggs

1½ cup almond milk

2 tbsp. vegetable oil

Directions

1. Preheat waffle iron.

2. In a large bowl, mix together flour, baking powder, stevia.

3. In a separate bowl, mix eggs, milk, oil, lemon juice and vanilla extract.

4. Pour liquid mixture into soft ingredients. Mix just until blended.

5. Let batter rest for 5

2 tsp. lemon juice

3 tsp. vanilla extract.

minutes.

6. Ladle batter onto waffle iron and cook until golden a crisp.

Banana Oat Shake

Prep time: 10 min | Cooking time: 0 min | Servings: 2

NUTRITION PER SERVING:

Calories: 172 | Carbs: 33g | Protein: 6g | Fats: 4g | Phosphorus: 160mg | Potassium: 297mg | Sodium: 42mg.

Ingredients

½ cup cooked oatmeal, cold

⅔ cup almond milk

1 tbsp. stevia

1 tbsp. wheat germ

1½ tsp. vanilla extract

½ frozen banana, chunks.

Directions

1. Place oatmeal in blender and blend for a few minutes.

2. Add milk, brown sugar, wheat germ, vanilla, and 1/2 banana. Blend until thick and smooth.

Sweet Broiled Grapefruit

Prep time: 5 min | Cooking time: 10 min | Servings: 2

NUTRITION PER SERVING:

Calories: 203 | Fat: 12g | Saturated Fat: 7g | Cholesterol: 31mg | Sodium: 116mg | Carbohydrate: 26g | Sugars: 24g | Fiber: 2g | Protein: 1g.

Ingredients

1 large grapefruit

2 tbsp. butter, softened

2 tbsp. sugar

½ tsp. ground cinnamon.

Directions

1. Preheat broiler. Cut around each grapefruit section to loosen fruit. Top with butter. Mix sugar and cinnamon, sprinkle over fruit.

2. Place on a baking sheet. Broil 4 in. from heat until sugar is bubbly.

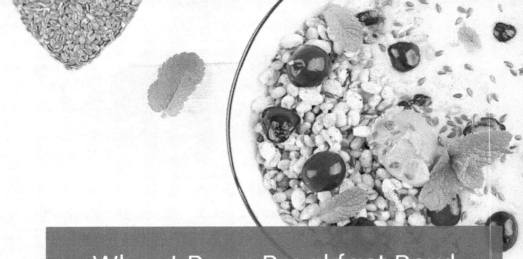

Wheat Berry Breakfast Bowl

Prep time: 20 min | Cooking time: 1 h | Servings: 4

NUTRITION PER SERVING:

Calories 174 | Fat 2g | Sodium 19mg| Potassium 220mg | Carbohydrates 36g | Protein 3g | Phosphorus 90mg.

Ingredients

½ cups wheat berries, uncooked

1½ cup water

1 medium fresh pear

1 tbsp. unsalted butter

½ cup fresh cranberries

2 tbsp. crystallized ginger

Directions

1. To cook wheat berries, bring water and wheat berries to a boil. Turn down heat to simmer and put lid on pan. Simmer for 30 minutes.

2. Check for doneness and add extra water if needed. Continue cooking for 15-20 minutes, checking every 5 minutes until done. Wheat berries

1 tsp. fresh orange zest

2 tbsp. maple syrup

½ tsp. cinnamon.

should be al dente or chewy.

1. Thinly slice pear. Heat butter in sauté pan and add pear slices. Cook until tender.

2. Add cranberries and chopped crystallized ginger to pears. Cook until cranberries start to burst.

3. Add cooked wheat berries, orange zest, maple syrup and cinnamon. Stir until heated through. Serve and enjoy!

Notes: Cook wheat berries the day before and refrigerate until ready to use. Add a vegetable milk if desired. Substitute 1/4 cup dried cranberries if fresh are not available.

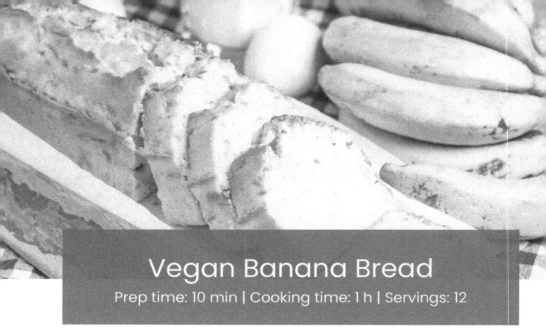

Vegan Banana Bread

Prep time: 10 min | Cooking time: 1 h | Servings: 12

NUTRITION PER SERVING:

Calories 200 | Fat 7g | Sodium 111mg| Potassium 223mg | Carbohydrates 23g | Protein 3g | Phosphorus 78mg.

Ingredients

4 medium bananas, ripe

⅓ cup vegetable oil

½ cup stevia

⅛ tsp. salt

½ cup applesauce

1½ tsp. vanilla extract

4 tbsp. flax seeds, ground

Directions

4. Preheat the oven to 350°F.

5. Peel the bananas and mash with a fork. Place in a mixing bowl.

6. Mix the vegetable oil into the mashed bananas with a wooden spoon.

7. Add and stir in stevia, salt, applesauce, vanilla, ground flaxseeds, baking soda, and agave nectar

1 tsp. sodium free baking soda

2 tbsp. agave nectar

1½ cup all-purpose white flour.

into the bowl.

8. Add the flour. Stir until ingredients are well incorporated. Pour into a greased 9x5-inch loaf pan.

9. Bake 50-60 minutes, or until the top springs back slightly depressed. Cool on a rack.

Pumpkin Spiced Bread with Applesauce

Prep time: 10 min | Cooking time: 50 min | Servings: 12

NUTRITION PER SERVING:

Calories 232 | Fat 2.6g | Sodium 121mg | Carbohydrates 28g | Dietary Fiber 9g | Protein 3g | Potassium 82mg | Phosphorus 41mg.

This moist bread gives you the softness of applesauce with the crisp spices of pumpkin pie for a sweet breakfast or snack.

Ingredients

1½ cup unsweetened applesauce

½ cup stevia

½ cup vegetable oil

2 eggs

2 cups all-purpose

Directions

1. Preheat oven to 350°F.

2. Grease loaf.

3. In a medium bowl, whisk applesauce, stevia, oil, and eggs together.

4. In a separate medium bowl, mix remaining

white flour

1 tsp. sodium free baking soda

½ tsp. sodium-free baking powder

2 tsp. pumpkin pie spice.

ingredients.

5. Add applesauce mixture to flour mixture and stir until just combined (careful not to over mix).

6. Place batter in loaf.

7. Bake for about 50-60 minutes. You can test doneness by poking with a toothpick, which should come out clean.

Cornbread

Prep time: 10 min | Cooking time: 60 min | Servings: 8

NUTRITION PER SERVING:

Calories: 166 | Carbs: 35g | Protein: 5g | Fats: 1g | Phosphorus: 79mg | Potassium: 122mg | Sodium: 34mg.

Ingredients

2 tbsps. shortening

1¼ cups skim milk

¼ cup egg substitute

4 tbsps. sodium free baking powder

½ cup white flour

1½ cups cornmeal.

Directions

1. Preheat the oven to 425°F.

2. In a large bowl, mix the cornmeal, baking powder and baking powder.

3. In medium bowl, whisk the eggs until foamy. Whisk in the milk.

4. Make a well in the center of the dry ingredients. Add the wet ingredients to the dry ingredients and mix until just blended.

5. Prepare 8 x 8-inch baking dish and add shortening. Put the baking dish in the oven for 5 minutes or until the shortening has

melted.

6. Remove the baking dish from the oven, and immediately pour in the batter. Stir well. Once done, pour the mixture into baking dish.

7. Return the baking dish to the oven, and bake for 15 to 20 minutes, or until the top is golden and the center is just cooked through. Taking care not to over-bake will ensure moist cornbread.

8. Serve hot or at room temperature.

Notes: Wrap tightly and refrigerate any leftovers. If the leftovers become dry, wrap lightly in a damp paper towel and reheat gently in the microwave. This will "refresh" the cornbread.

Scrambled Veggie Eggs

Prep time: 5 min | Cooking time: 7 min | Servings: 2

NUTRITION PER SERVING:

Calories 240 | Total Fat 16.6g | Cholesterol 372mg | Sodium 195mg | Total Carbohydrate 7.8g | Dietary Fiber 2.7g | Protein 15.3g | Potassium 605.2mg | Phosphorus 203.6mg.

This is a great basic recipe for increasing your vegetable intake!

Ingredients

2 whole eggs

4 egg whites

1 cup cauliflower

3 cup fresh spinach

1 garlic clove, minced

¼ cup bell pepper, chopped

¼ cup onion, chopped

¼ tsp. black pepper

Directions

1. Beat eggs with pepper until light and fluffy, set aside.

2. Heat oil over medium heat in large skillet.

3. Add onions and peppers to skillet and sauté until peppers are translucent and golden.

4. Add garlic, stirring quickly to combine and immediately adding cauliflower and spinach.

1 tbsp. oil of choice (coconut or avocado oil is good for high heat)

Fresh parsley and spring onion for garnish.

5. Sauté vegetables, turn heat to medium-low and cover for 5 minutes.

6. Add eggs, stirring to combine with vegetables.

7. When the eggs are cooked thoroughly, top with fresh parsley or spring onions.

Notes: Other spices/herbs that would be delicious with this include herbs de Provence, red pepper flakes, extra garlic, and basil. You can also add a little of lemon juice to your eggs to bring out the flavors rather than using salt.

To reduce phosphorus further you can you 8 egg whites instead of egg yolks.

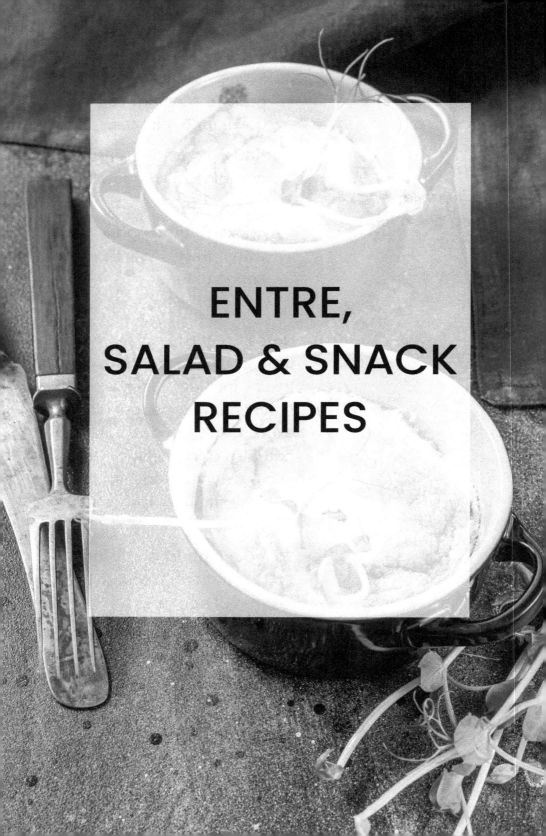

ENTRE, SALAD & SNACK RECIPES

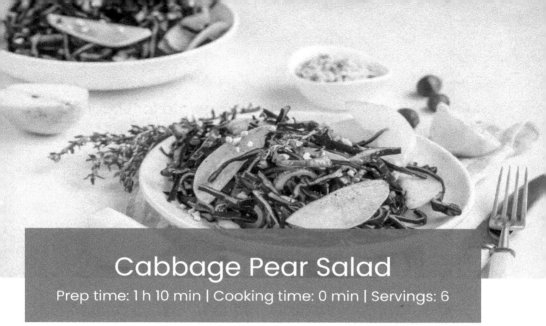

Cabbage Pear Salad

Prep time: 1 h 10 min | Cooking time: 0 min | Servings: 6

NUTRITION PER SERVING:

Calories: 128 | Fat: 8g | Phosphorus: 25mg | Potassium: 149mg | Sodium: 57mg | Carbs: 2g | Protein: 6g.

Ingredients

2 scallions, chopped

2 cups green cabbage, finely shredded

1 cup red cabbage, finely shredded

½ red bell pepper, boiled and chopped

½ cup cilantro,

Directions

1. In a mixing bowl, add cabbages, scallions, celery, pear, red pepper, and cilantro. Combine to mix well with each other.

2. Take another mixing bowl; add olive oil, lime juice, lime zest, and stevia. Combine to mix well with each other.

3. Add dressing over and

chopped

2 celery stalks, chopped

1 Asian pear, cored and grated

¼ cup olive oil

1 lime fresh juice

1 lime zest

½ tsp. stevia.

toss well.

4. Refrigerate for 1 hour.

5. Serve chilled.

Arugula Parmesan Salad

Prep time: 10 min | Cooking time: 0 min | Servings:4

NUTRITION PER SERVING:

Calories: 61 | Fat: 4g | Phosphorus: 34mg | Potassium: 53mg | Sodium: 55mg | Carbs: 1g | Protein: 2g.

Ingredients

2 cups arugula, loosely packed

1 tbsp. extra-virgin olive oil

1 shallot, thinly sliced

3 celery stalks

2 tbsp. white wine vinegar

Black pepper, to taste

2 tbsp. Parmesan cheese.

Directions

1. Cut celery stalks into 1-inch pieces about ¼ inch thick.

2. In a mixing bowl, add shallot, celery stalks, and arugula. Combine to mix well with each other.

3. Take another mixing bowl; add olive oil, vinegar, and black pepper. Combine to mix well with each other. Add dressing over and toss well. Grate Parmesan cheese on top and serve fresh.

Broccoli & Apple Salad

Prep time: 15 min | Cooking time: 0 min | Servings: 8

NUTRITION PER SERVING:

Calories 160 | Carbs 18g | Protein 4g | Fat 8g | Sodium 63mg | Potassium 220mg | Phosphorous 74mg.

Ingredients

¾ cup low-fat Greek yogurt

¼ cup mayonnaise

2 tbsp. honey

2 tbsp. apple cider vinegar

4 cups fresh broccoli florets

1 medium apple

½ cup red onion

¼ cup fresh parsley

½ cup dried cranberries

¼ cup walnuts.

Directions

1. Trim and cut broccoli florets into small bite size pieces. Dice unpeeled apple into small bite size pieces. Chop the fresh parsley.

2. In a large bowl whisk together the yogurt, mayonnaise, honey, vinegar and parsley.

3. Add the remaining ingredients and coat with the yogurt mixture. Refrigerate to chill and let the flavors combine. Stir immediately before serving.

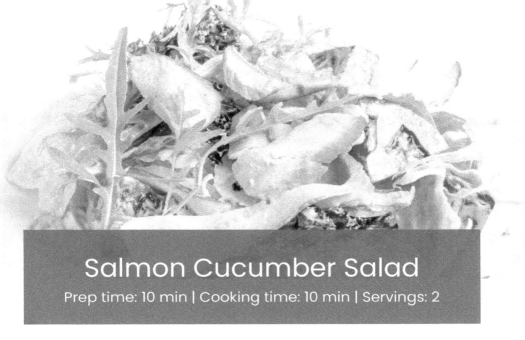

Salmon Cucumber Salad

Prep time: 10 min | Cooking time: 10 min | Servings: 2

NUTRITION PER SERVING:

Calories: 288 | Fat: 14g | Phosphorus: 217mg | Potassium: 548mg | Sodium: 178mg | Carbohydrates: 17g | Protein: 26g.

Ingredients

1 cup fennel bulb, diced

1 cup red onions, diced

½ lb. salmon fillets

1 cup cucumber, peeled, diced

2 tbsp. + 1 tsp. olive oil

3 tbsp. apple cider vinegar

Directions

1. Preheat an oven to 400°F. Grease a baking dish with 1 teaspoon olive oil. Season salmon with black pepper with skin side down. Placed over the baking dish, bake for 8-10 minutes until easy to flake.

2. In bowl, whisk vinegar and remaining oil.

3. Flake salmon and add it

Black pepper, to taste.

in a bowl. Add remaining ingredients and combine well. Serve fresh.

Kale Slaw

Prep time: 35 min | Cooking time: 0 min | Servings: 6

NUTRITION PER SERVING:

Calories: 143 | Fat: 7g | Phosphorus: 38mg | Potassium: 245mg | Sodium: 29mg | Carbs: 18g | Protein: 2g.

Ingredients

½ bunch fresh kale

2 tbsp. shallots

6 medium Brussels sprouts

⅓ cup dried, sweetened cranberries

3 tbsp. olive oil

3 tbsp. cider vinegar

3 tbsp. honey

1 tsp. garlic & herb seasoning blend

½ tsp. yellow mustard

⅛ tsp. black pepper.

Directions

1. Remove kale from stalks and finely chop. Measure 3 cups for slaw. Chop shallots.

2. Shred Brussels sprouts and measure 2 cups.

3. In a medium bowl, combine kale, Brussels sprouts, cranberries and shallots.

4. In a small bowl, combine olive oil, vinegar, honey, seasoning blend, mustard and pepper. Pour over vegetables and mix.

5. Refrigerate for 30 minutes before serving.

Notes: Kale slaw keeps in the refrigerator for 5 days.

For a variation, heat the slaw and stir-fry for a hot dish.

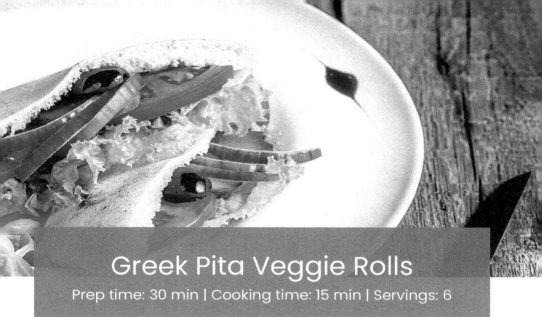

Greek Pita Veggie Rolls

Prep time: 30 min | Cooking time: 15 min | Servings: 6

NUTRITION PER SERVING:

Calories: 120 | Fat: 2.8g | Carbs: 20.7g | Fiber: 1.5g | Protein: 3.3g | Potassium: 156mg | Sodium: 164mg.

Ingredients

1 cup romaine lettuce, shredded

1 red bell pepper, seeded and chopped

½ cup cucumber, chopped

1 small tomato, seeded and chopped

1 small red onion,

Directions

1. In a large bowl, add all ingredients except pita breads and gently toss to coat well.

2. Arrange pita breads onto serving plates.

3. Place veggie mixture in the center of each pita bread evenly.

4. Roll the pita bread and serve.

chopped

1 garlic clove, finely minced

1 tbsp. olive oil

½ tbsp. fresh lemon juice

Freshly ground black pepper, to taste

3 (6½-inch) pita breads.

Crispy Kale Chips

Prep time: 10 min | Cooking time: 15 min | Servings: 6

NUTRITION PER SERVING:

Calories 28 | Carbs: 2g | Protein: 1g | Fats: 3g | Phosphorus: 15mg | Potassium: 79mg | Sodium: 394mg.

Ingredients

1 tbsp. olive oil

1 tsp. salt

6 cups kale, torn.

Directions

1. With cooking spray, lightly grease the baking sheet. Preheat oven to 350°F.

2. Remove the kale leaves from its stems and tear into bite-sized pieces. Place kale on the prepped baking sheet. Drizzle with olive oil and season with salt. Toss kale leaves to coat well with oil and salt.

3. Pop into the oven and bake for 10 to 15 minutes or until leaf edges are turning brown but not burnt.

Steamed Zucchini

Prep time: 5 min | Cooking time: 15 min | Servings: 2

NUTRITION PER SERVING:

Calories 64 | Sodium 20mg | Carbs 7.1g | Protein 2.5g | Potassium 117mg | Phosphorus 101mg.

Ingredients

2 zucchini

2 cloves garlic

1 tbsp. olive oil.

Directions

1. Bring a large pot of water to a boil. Trim ends from zucchini. Place zucchini and garlic into a steamer basket, then place the steamer basket into the pot. Steam for 10 to 15 minutes, or until the zucchini are tender.

1. Transfer zucchini to a large bowl. Mash the garlic and put it in the bowl with the zucchini. Drizzle the olive oil into the bowl and toss until the vegetables are coated with oil and garlic.

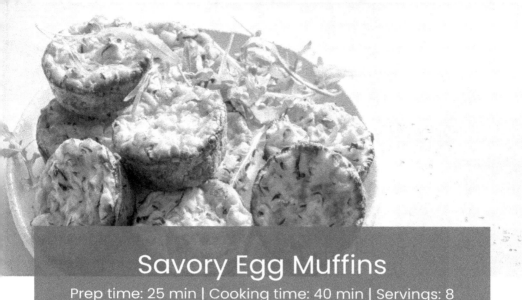

Savory Egg Muffins

Prep time: 25 min | Cooking time: 40 min | Servings: 8

NUTRITION PER SERVING:

Calories 154 | Fat 10g | Sodium 155mg | Carbs 3g | Protein 12g | Potassium 200mg | Phosphorus 154mg.

Ingredients

1 cup bell peppers (red, yellow, and orange)

1 cup onion

½ lb. ground pork

¼ tsp. poultry seasoning

¼ tsp. garlic powder

¼ tsp. onion powder

Directions

1. Preheat oven to 350°F and spray a regular size muffin tin with cooking spray.

1. Finely dice bell peppers and onion.

2. In a bowl combine pork, poultry seasoning, garlic powder, onion powder and Italian herbs seasoning to make

½ tsp. Italian herbs seasoning blend

8 large eggs

2 tbsp. soy milk

1/4 tsp. salt (optional).

3. In a nonstick skillet, cook sausage crumbles until done; drain.

4. Beat eggs together with the milk and salt.

5. Add the sausage crumbles and vegetables, mix.

6. Pour egg mixture into prepared muffin tins, leaving space for muffins to rise. Bake for 18 to 22 minutes.

Notes: To reduce phosphorus further you can you 16 egg whites instead of egg yolks.

Deviled Eggs

Prep time: 10 min | Cooking time: 10 min | Servings: 2

NUTRITION PER SERVING:

Calories 90 | Carbs 1g | Protein 6g | Potassium 94mg | Phosphorous 34mg.

Ingredients

2 large eggs, hard-boiled

2 tsp. canned pimento

2 tbsp. low sodium mayo

½ tsp. black pepper

¼ tsp. paprika

½ tsp. dry mustard.

Directions

1. Cut the eggs lengthwise in half and remove the yolk.

1. Mix the egg yolk with the dry mustard, mayonnaise, and black pepper.

2. Pile the mixture back into the egg whites.

3. Sprinkle with paprika and serve.

Creamy Cucumber Spread

Prep time: 10 min | Cooking time: 0 min | Servings: 8

NUTRITION PER SERVING:

Calories 115 | Fat 8g | Carbs 2g | Protein 2g | Sodium 100mg | Potassium 73mg | Phosphorous 36mg.

Ingredients

8 oz. low-fat or fat-free cream cheese

1 medium cucumber

1 tsp. onion

1 tbsp. low-sodium mayonnaise.

Directions

1. Peel, seed and finely mince cucumber. Mince onion.

2. Mix cream cheese, onion and mayonnaise in a small bowl and blend until smooth.

3. Fold cucumber into mixture until evenly blended.

Salmon Sandwich

Prep time: 10 min | Cooking time: 12 min | Servings: 4

NUTRITION PER SERVING:

Calories 382 | Protein 26g | Sodium 384mg | Potassium 640mg | Phosphorus 268mg | Fiber 1.0g.

Ingredients

2 tbsp. olive oil, divided

1 tbsp. lime juice

½ tsp. lemon-pepper seasoning

4 salmon fillets

¼ cup chipotle mayonnaise

4 slices white bread

1 cup arugula

2 roasted red peppers, diced.

Directions

1. Preheat your grill.

1. Coat salmon with half of the oil. Grill for 12 minutes.

2. In a bowl, mix the oil, lime juice, and lemon pepper seasoning.

3. Toast the bread in the grill.

4. Spread mayo on the bread and arrange arugula and roasted red peppers. Place salmon on top.

Fresh Tofu Spring Rolls

Prep time: 35 min | Cooking time: 5 min | Servings: 6

NUTRITION PER SERVING:

Calories 156 | Fat 5g | Sodium 161mg | Carbs 20g | Protein 8g | Potassium 302mg | Phosphorus 93mg.

Ingredients

12 leaves Romaine lettuce

2 medium carrots

½ medium red onion

16 oz. firm tofu

½ tbsp. ground cumin

½ tbsp. granulated garlic

¼ tsp. sea salt

½ tsp. black pepper

1 tbsp. olive oil

12 rice wrappers for spring rolls.

Directions

1. Wash and dry the lettuce, then cut each leaf in half lengthwise. Cut carrots julienne style. Slice onion.

2. Drain and pat dry the tofu. Slice it into 12 pieces, each about 4-inch long.

3. Spread the tofu on plate and season it evenly with cumin, granulated garlic, sea salt and black pepper.

4. Heat a non-stick pan with olive oil. Place the tofu strips in the pan, seasoned side down. Season the other side and fry until the bottom is

lightly browned, about 1 to 2 minutes. Flip and fry until second side is lightly browned. Let cool.

5. Boil 6 cups of water. Pour it into a large shallow bowl. Dip a rice wrapper in.

6. Once it's slightly soft, place the wrapper on a large plate and place 2 halves of the lettuce in the center of the wrapper. Sprinkle 2 to 3 tablespoons of carrot and 1- to 2 tablespoons of sliced onion on top of the lettuce. Place one cooled tofu strip on top of the vegetables.

7. Fold the sides in, and then fold the bottom up and roll tightly. Repeat with the rest of the rice wrappers, vegetables and tofu strips.

8. Refrigerate and serve cold with your favorite

low-sodium dressing.

Notes: Serve with 2 tablespoons of low-sodium dressing. Miso ginger dressing is a good choice.

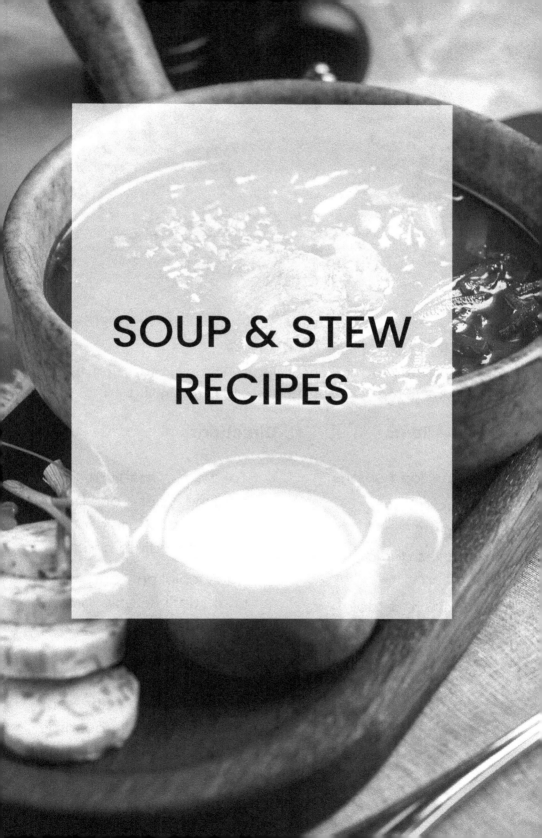

SOUP & STEW RECIPES

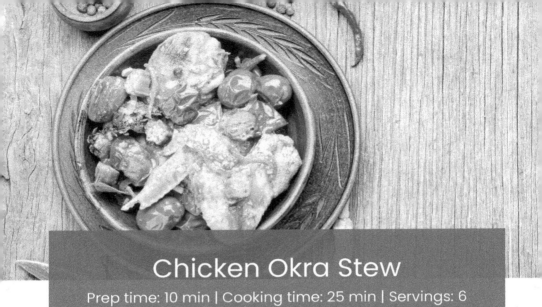

Chicken Okra Stew

Prep time: 10 min | Cooking time: 25 min | Servings: 6

NUTRITION PER SERVING:

Calories: 153 | Fat: 8g | Phosphorus: 135mg | Potassium: 469mg
| Sodium: 110mg | Carbohydrates: 14g | Protein: 10g.

Ingredients

1 cup sliced onions

¾ cup green peppers

2 cloves garlic, minced

3 tbsp. vegetable oil

2 lb. chicken breasts, cut into bite-sized pieces

1 10-ounce bag

Directions

1. Take a medium-large cooking pot or Dutch oven, heat 2 tablespoons oil over medium heat.

1. Add chicken and stir-cook until evenly brown. Set aside.

2. Add 1 tablespoon oil. Add onion, garlic, green peppers, and stir-cook until they become softened. Add flour and

frozen carrots

¼ tsp. dried basil

¼ tsp. black pepper

2 tbsp. all-purpose flour

2 (10.5-ounce) cans low-sodium chicken broth

6 lb. sliced okra.

stir-cook for 2-3 minutes.

3. Add broth, chicken, and boil the mixture.

4. Add carrots, black pepper, and basil.

5. Over low heat, cover, and simmer the mixture for about 10-15 minutes until gravy thickens.

6. Add okra and cook for 5-10 minutes more until tender.

7. Serve with cooked white rice (optional).

Cabbage Turkey Soup

Prep time: 10 min | Cooking time: 45 min | Servings: 6

NUTRITION PER SERVING:

Calories: 83 | Fat: 4g | Phosphorus: 91mg | Potassium: 185mg | Sodium: 63mg | Carbs: 2g | Protein: 8g.

Cozy up with this savory turkey and cabbage soup – tender turkey beats, mixed vegetables simmered in a rich homemade-broth. Grain-free, minimal ingredients, and super tasty!

Ingredients

½ cup green cabbage, shredded

½ cup bulgur

2 dried bay leaves

2 tbsp. fresh parsley, finely chopped

1 tsp. fresh sage,

Directions

1. Take a large saucepan or cooking pot, add oil. Heat over medium heat.

2. Add turkey and stir-cook for 4-5 minutes until evenly brown.

3. Add onion and garlic and sauté for about 3 minutes to soften veggies.

chopped

1 tsp. fresh thyme, chopped

1 celery stalk, chopped

1 carrot, sliced thin

½ sweet onion, chopped

1 tsp. garlic, minced

1 tsp. olive oil

½ lb. cooked ground turkey, 93% lean

4 cups water

1 cup chicken stock

Pinch red pepper flakes

Ground black pepper, to taste.

4. Add water, chicken stock, cabbage, bulgur, celery, carrot, and bay leaves.

5. Boil the mixture.

6. Over low heat, cover, and simmer the mixture for about 30-35 minutes until bulgur is cooked well and tender.

7. Remove bay leaves. Add parsley, sage, thyme, and red pepper flakes. Stir mixture and season with black pepper.

8. Serve warm.

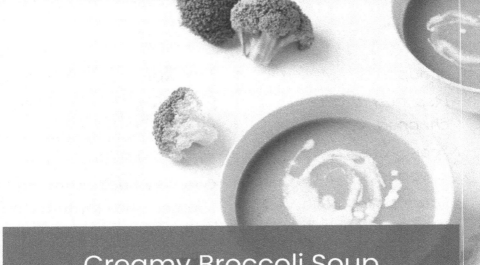

Creamy Broccoli Soup

Prep time: 10 min | Cooking time: 45 min | Servings: 5

NUTRITION PER SERVING:

Calories 65 | Carbs 10g | Protein 4g | Fat 1g | Sodium 71mg | Potassium 289mg | Phosphorous 90mg.

Ingredients

2 cups low-sodium vegetable broth

3 cups broccoli florets

8 oz. silken tofu, undrained

3 tbps. cornstarch

3 tbsp. nutritional yeast

Directions

1. In a large pot, boil the broccoli florets and tofu (with liquid) in the vegetable broth until tender. Set aside to cool.

2. Carefully pour the cooled contents of the pot into a large mixing bowl and blend until smooth using an immersion blender. Alternately, carefully pour

1 tsp. onion powder

1 tsp. garlic powder

¼ tsp. black pepper

⅛ tsp. red pepper flakes.

contents of the pot into a large blender. Remove top stopper to allow steam to vent. Blend until smooth.

3. In a small bowl, combine 1-1/2 cups of the soup with the cornstarch. Whisk until smooth.

4. Pour soup back into the pot, add cornstarch mixture and bring to a boil. Stir in nutritional yeast and spices until well combined.

Beef Okra Soup

Prep time: 10 min | Cooking time: 45 min | Servings: 5

NUTRITION PER SERVING:

Calories: 187 | Fat: 12g | Phosphorus: 119mg | Potassium: 288mg | Sodium: 59mg | Carbs: 7g | Protein: 11g.

Ingredients

½ cup okra

½ tsp. basil

½ cup carrots, diced

3½ cups water

1 lb. beef stew meat

1 cup raw onions, sliced

½ cup green peas

1 tsp. black pepper

½ tsp. thyme

½ cup corn kernels.

Directions

1. Take a medium-large cooking pot, heat oil over medium heat.

1. Add water, beef stew meat, black pepper, onions, basil, thyme, and stir-cook for ,40-45 minutes until meat is tender.

2. Add all veggies. Over low heat, simmer the mixture for about 20-25 minutes. Add more water if needed.

3. Serve soup warm.

Roasted Red Pepper Soup

Prep time: 30 min | Cooking time: 35 min | Servings: 4

NUTRITION PER SERVING:

Calories 266 | Fat 8g | Fiber 6g | Carbs 15g | Protein 3g | Sodium 225mg | Potassium 455mg.

Ingredients

4 cups chicken broth

3 red peppers

2 medium onions

1 lemon juice and zest

A pinch cayenne pepper

¼ tsp. cinnamon

½ cup fresh cilantro, minced.

Directions

1. In a medium stockpot, consolidate each one of the fixings except for the cilantro and warmth to the point of boiling over excessive warm temperature.

2. Diminish the warmth and stew, ordinarily secured, for around 30 minutes, till thickened. Cool marginally.

3. Utilizing a hand blender or nourishment processor, puree the soup. Include the cilantro and tenderly heat.

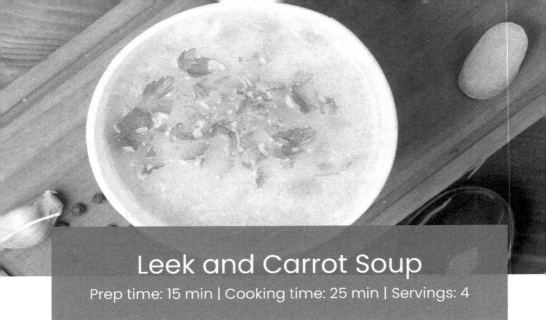

Leek and Carrot Soup

Prep time: 15 min | Cooking time: 25 min | Servings: 4

NUTRITION PER SERVING:

Calories 325 | Fat 9g | Carbs 16g | Protein 29g | Sodium 301mg | Potassium 150mg | Phosphorous 22mg.

Ingredients

1 tbsp. oil

2 leeks, chopped

2 celery stalks, chopped

1 garlic clove

3 carrots, diced

Crushed pepper to taste

3 cups low-sodium vegetable broth

Directions

1. In a large stove pot, heat oil over medium heat for 1 minute.

2. Add chopped leeks, celery and garlic. Stir-cook for 2-3 minutes, until become translucent and softened. Add carrots, stirring continuously, cook until carrots are slightly tender, about 5 minutes.

3. Pour vegetable broth into

1 bay leaf

¼ tsp. ground cumin

Chopped parsley for garnish.

the pot; add bay leaf and pepper. Bring the mixture to a boil and cook over medium-low heat for 10-15 minutes. Remove from heat. Remove and discard bay leaf.

4. Using an immersion blender, blend together to reach desired consistency. Add more water if desired.

5. Stir in cumin if using, garnish with chopped parsley, and serve hot.

Notes: Other spices that go well with leeks are tarragon, thyme, and sage. To make it spicy, add red pepper flakes!

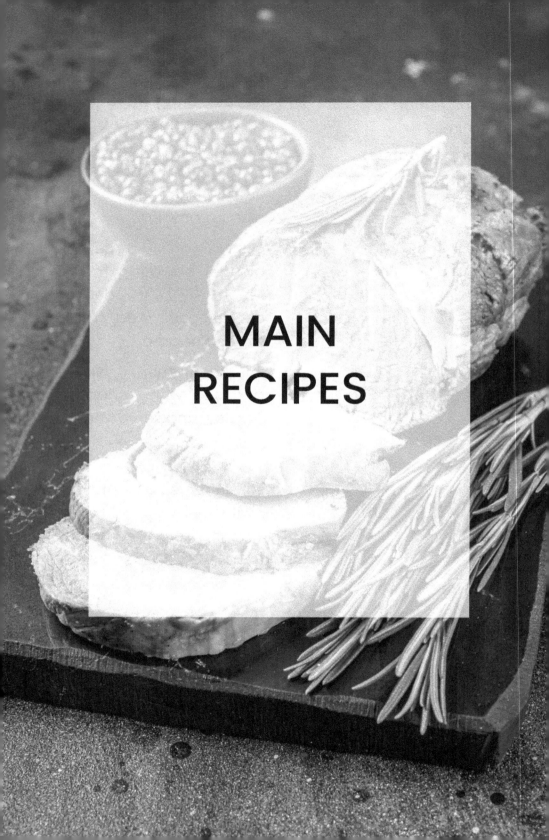

MAIN
RECIPES

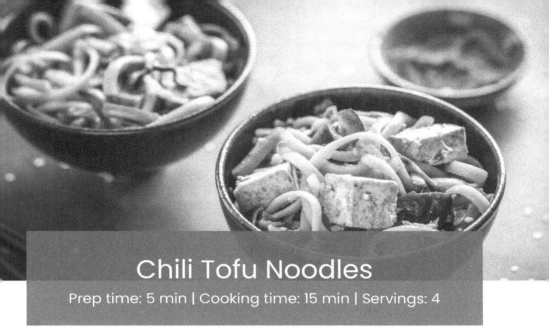

Chili Tofu Noodles

Prep time: 5 min | Cooking time: 15 min | Servings: 4

NUTRITION PER SERVING:

Calories 246 | Protein 10g | Carbs 28g | Fat 12g | Sodium 25mg | Potassium 126mg | Phosphorus 79mg.

Ingredients

½ red chili, diced

2 cups rice noodles

½ juiced lime

6 oz. silken firm tofu, pressed and cubed

1 tsp. fresh ginger, grated

1 tbsp. coconut oil

1 cup green beans

Directions

1. Steam the green beans for 10-12 minutes or according to package directions and drain.

1. Cook the noodles in a pot of boiling water for 10-15 minutes or according to package directions.

2. Meanwhile, heat a wok or skillet on high heat and add coconut oil.

1 garlic clove, minced.

3. Now add the tofu, chili flakes, garlic, and ginger and sauté for 5-10 minutes.

4. After doing that, drain in the noodles along with the green beans and lime juice, then add it to the wok.

5. Toss to coat.

6. Serve hot!

Elegant Veggie Tortillas

Prep time: 30 min | Cooking time: 15 min | Servings: 12

NUTRITION PER SERVING:

Calories: 217 | Fat: 3.3g | Carbs: 41g | Protein: 8.1g | Fiber: 6.3g | Potassium: 289mg | Sodium: 87mg.

Veggie corn tortillas are super healthy, kidney friendly, easy to make and perfect for lunch or dinner.

Ingredients

1½ cups broccoli florets, chopped

1½ cups cauliflower florets, chopped

1 tbsp. water

2 tsp. canola oil

1½ cups onion, chopped

1 garlic clove, minced

2 tbsp. fresh parsley, finely

Directions

1. In a microwave bowl, place broccoli, cauliflower, and water and microwave, covered for about 3-5 minutes.

2. Remove from the microwave and drain any liquid.

3. Heat oil on medium heat.

4. Add onion and sauté for about 4-5 minutes.

5. Add garlic and then sauté

chopped

1 cup low-sodium liquid egg substitute

Freshly ground black pepper, to taste

4 (6-ounce) warmed corn tortillas.

it for about 1 minute.

6. Stir in broccoli, cauliflower, parsley, egg substitute, and black pepper.

7. Reduce the heat and it to simmer for about 10 minutes.

8. Remove from heat and keep aside to cool slightly.

9. Place broccoli mixture over ¼ of each tortilla.

10. Fold the outside edges inward and roll up like a burrito.

11. Secure each tortilla with toothpicks to secure the filling.

12. Cut each tortilla in half and serve.

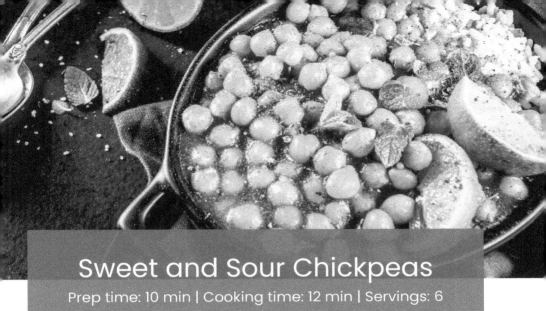

Sweet and Sour Chickpeas

Prep time: 10 min | Cooking time: 12 min | Servings: 6

NUTRITION PER SERVING:

Calories: 333 | Sodium: 15mg | Phosphorus: 253mg | Potassium: 505mg | Protein: 13g.

Ingredients

2 tbsp. extra-virgin olive oil

1 onion, chopped

1 (14-ounce) can tropical fruit in fruit juice, strained, reserving juice

2 tbsp. freshly squeezed lemon juice

2 tbsp. cornstarch

Directions

1. In a large saucepan, heat the olive oil over medium heat.

2. Cook the onion for 4 to 5 minutes, stirring frequently, until tender.

3. In a medium bowl, whisk together the fruit juice, lemon juice, and cornstarch.

4. When the onion is tender,

2 (15-ounce) cans no-salt-added chickpeas, drained and rinsed.

add the chickpeas and cook for 3 to 4 minutes, stirring until hot.

5. Add the juice mixture and cook, stirring frequently, until the liquid is thickened, about 2 minutes.

6. Add the drained fruits to the saucepan and simmer for 1 to 2 minutes or until hot.

7. Serve warm.

Cabbage-Stuffed Mushrooms

Prep time: 20 min | Cooking time: 25 min | Servings: 6

NUTRITION PER SERVING:

Calories: 163 | Sodium: 179mg | Phosphorus: 173mg | Potassium: 360mg | Protein: 7g.

Ingredients

6 Portobello mushrooms

3 tbsp. extra-virgin olive oil

1 onion, chopped

1 tsp. fresh ginger, peeled, minced

2 cups red cabbage, shredded

⅛ tsp. salt

⅛ tsp. freshly ground black pepper

3 tbsp. water

1 cup Monterey Jack cheese, shredded.

Directions

1. Rinse the mushrooms briefly and pat dry.

2. Remove the stems and discard.

3. Using a spoon, scrape out the dark gills on the underside of the mushroom cap. Set aside.

1. In a medium skillet, heat the olive oil over medium heat.

2. Cook the onion and ginger for 2 to 3 minutes, stirring until fragrant.

3. Add the cabbage, salt, and pepper and sauté for 3 minutes, stirring

frequently.

4. Add the water, cover, and steam the cabbage for 3 to 4 minutes, or until it is tender.

5. Remove the vegetables from the skillet and place in a medium bowl.

6. Let cool for 10 minutes, then stir in the cheese.

7. Preheat the oven to 400°F.

8. Place the caps on a baking sheet and divide the filling among the mushrooms.

9. Bake for 15 to 17 minutes, or until the mushrooms are tender and the filling is light golden brown.

10. Serve hot.

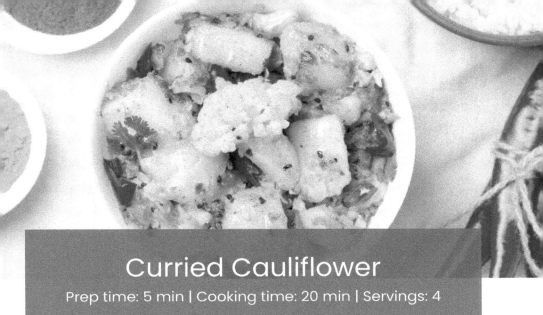

Curried Cauliflower

Prep time: 5 min | Cooking time: 20 min | Servings: 4

NUTRITION PER SERVING:

Calories 108 | Protein 2g | Carbs 11g | Fat 7g | Sodium 35mg | Potassium 328mg | Phosphorus 39mg.

Ingredients

1 tsp. turmeric

1 onion, diced

1 tbsp. fresh cilantro, chopped

1 tsp. cumin

½ chili, diced

½ cup water

1 garlic clove, minced

1 tbsp. coconut oil

1 tsp. gram

Directions

1. Add the oil to a skillet on medium heat.

2. Sauté the onion and garlic for 5 minutes until soft.

3. Add in the cumin, turmeric, and gram masala and stir to release the aromas.

4. Now add the chili to the pan along with the

masala

2 cups cauliflower florets.

cauliflower. Stir to coat.

5. Pour in the water and reduce the heat to a simmer for 15 minutes.

6. Garnish with cilantro to serve.

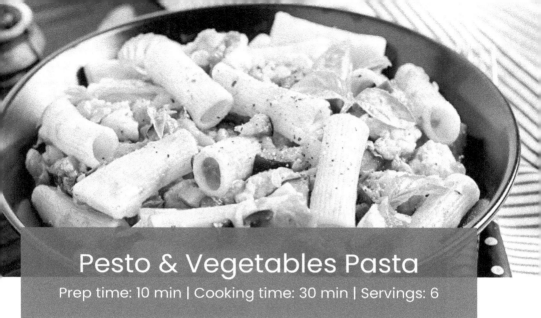

Pesto & Vegetables Pasta

Prep time: 10 min | Cooking time: 30 min | Servings: 6

NUTRITION PER SERVING:

Calories: 492 | Sodium: 336mg | Phosphorus: 237mg | Carbs: 66.9g | Potassium: 476mg | Protein: 13.4g | Fat 18.8g | Cholesterol 5.6mg.

Ingredients

16 oz. white pasta

2 medium zucchini, sliced into half moons

1 medium yellow squash, sliced into half moons

1 large red bell pepper, diced inch squares

½ cup mushrooms,

Directions

1. Preheat oven to 425°F.

1. Place zucchini, squash, bell pepper, onion and mushrooms on 18x13-inch baking sheet.

2. Drizzle veggies with olive oil then toss to evenly coat.

3. Roast in preheated oven until veggies tender,

sliced fairly thick

2 tbsp. olive oil

2 garlic cloves

⅔ cup pesto sauce

¼ cup feta cheese.

about 30 minutes.

4. While veggies are roasting cook pasta according to package and drain.

5. Pour drained pasta into a large bowl.

6. Add in roasted veggies and pesto then toss to evenly coat.

7. Serve warm.

Mexican Rice

Prep time: 10 min | Cooking time: 30 min | Servings: 6

NUTRITION PER SERVING:

Calories: 194 | Fat: 10g | Sodium: 94mg | Carbs: 24g | Protein: 2g | Potassium 77mg | Phosphorus 41mg.

Ingredients

¼ cup white onion, chopped

½ tsp. garlic, minced

¼ tsp. salt

¼ cup canola oil

¼ cup tomato sauce, low sodium

3 cups water

1 cup white rice, uncooked.

Directions

1. Take a medium-sized skillet pan, place it over medium-high heat, add oil and when hot, add rice and cook for 5 minutes until browned.

2. Then add onion and garlic, stir until mixed, and cook for 3 minutes, or until tender.

3. Season with salt, pour in tomato sauce and water, stir until mixed, simmer for 20 minutes until rice has cooked, covering the pan. Serve straight away.

Shrimp Fried Rice

Prep time: 5 min | Cooking time: 20 min | Servings: 4

NUTRITION PER SERVING:

Calories: 421 | Fat: 16 g | Sodium: 271mg | Carbs: 53g | Fiber: 2.5g | Protein: 16g | Potassium 285mg | Phosphorus 218mg.

Ingredients

4 cups white rice, cooked

½ cup small frozen shrimp, cooked

¾ cup white onion, chopped

1 cup frozen peas and carrots

3 tbsp. scallions, chopped

½ tsp. garlic, minced

1 tbsp. ginger root, grated

¼ tsp. salt

¾ tsp. ground black pepper

Directions

1. Take a large skillet pan, place it over medium-high heat, add 1 tablespoon peanut oil.

2. When hot, add onion, season with ½ teaspoon black pepper, and cook for 2 minutes, or until onions are tender.

3. Stir in scallions, ginger, and garlic, cook for 1 minute.

4. Add shrimps, stir until mixed, cook for 2 minutes until hot,

5. Then stir in carrots and peas and cook for 2

5 tbsp. peanut oil

4 eggs.

minutes until hot.

6. When done, transfer shrimps and vegetable mixture to a bowl, cover with a lid, and set aside until required.

7. Return the skillet pan over medium heat, add 2 tablespoons oil, beat the eggs, pour it into the pan, cook for 3 minutes until eggs are scrambled to the desired level, and then transfer eggs to the bowl containing shrimps and vegetables.

8. Add remaining 1 tablespoon oil, and when hot, add rice, stir until well coated, and cook for 2 minutes until hot.

9. Then season rice with salt and remaining black pepper, cook for 2 minutes, don't stir.

10. Then add eggs, shrimps, and vegetables, stir until mixed and cook for 3

minutes until hot.

11.   Serve straight away.

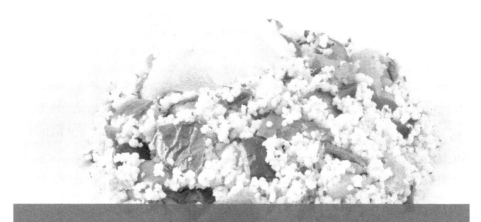

Lemon Couscous with Zucchini

Prep time: 10 min | Cooking time: 15 min | Servings: 5

NUTRITION PER SERVING:

Calories: 268 | Sodium: 19mg | Phosphorus: 78mg | Potassium: 187mg | Carbs: 48g | Protein: 5g | Fat 6g.

Ingredients

½ cup onion, chopped

½ cup celery, chopped

1 tbsp. parsley, finely chopped

½ cup zucchini

2 cups water

2 tbsp. canola oil

1 cup couscous, uncooked

Directions

1. Quarter and slice zucchini.

2. In a saucepan, combine the water and 1 tablespoon of the oil and bring to a boil. Stir in couscous and cover. Remove from heat; let stand 5 minutes.

3. Combine lemon juice with zest, cayenne pepper and

¼ cup lemon juice

2 tsp. lemon zest

¼ tsp. cayenne pepper

½ tsp. ground cumin

1 cup dried cranberries, sweetened.

cumin.

4. In a large skillet, heat remaining 1 tablespoon of canola oil over medium heat.

5. Sauté celery, onion and zucchini until softened.

6. Transfer into a large serving dish and mix together the cooked couscous, the vegetables, cranberries, parsley, lemon juice and seasonings.

7. Fluff with fork before serving.

8. Serve hot.

Veggie Burger

Prep time: 15 min | Cooking time: 30 min | Servings: 6

NUTRITION PER SERVING:

Calories: 145 | Sodium: 218mg | Phosphorus: 60mg | Potassium: 240mg | Carbs: 21.5g | Fat 5g | Protein: 4g.

Ingredients

2 cups cabbage, finely chopped

1 cup carrots, grated

2 cups frozen French style green beans, chopped

¼ tsp. salt

1 tsp. cumin powder

1 tsp. cilantro powder

1 tsp. red chili powder

½ cup all-purpose white flour

4 slices white bread

Directions

1. Soak bread slices in water and drain by squeezing between the palms of your hands.

2. In a medium pan cover cabbage and carrots with water and boil for 10 minutes.

3. Add the chopped green beans and cook until completely done.

4. Drain excess water and let cool.

5. Add spices, flour, bread slices, fresh cilantro and lime juice to vegetables and mix well.

*¼ cup fresh
cilantro, finely
chopped*

½ tsp. lime juice

2 tbsp. canola oil.

6. Make 12 balls and flatten each into a patty the size of a small burger.

7. Heat a saucepan over medium heat.

8. Add the oil and place patties in the saucepan, 2 or 3 at a time without crowding.

9. Flip patties over when cooked, about 2-3 minutes on each side.

10. Serve hot and enjoy!

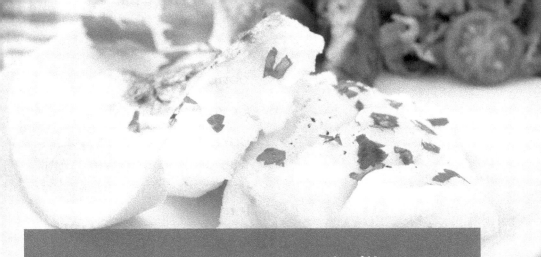

Lemon Butter Cod Fillet

Prep time: 20 min | Cooking time: 30 min | Servings: 5

NUTRITION PER SERVING:

Calories 168 | Sodium 210mg | Protein 6.7g | Potassium 29mg | Phosphorus 16mg.

Ingredients

½ cup butter

1 juiced lemon

1 tsp. ground black pepper

½ tsp. dried basil

3 garlic cloves, minced

6 (4-ounces) cod fillets

2 tbsp. lemon pepper.

Directions

1. Preheat oven to 350°F.

2. Arrange cod fillets in a single layer on a medium baking sheet.

3. Melt the butter in a medium saucepan over medium heat. Bring to a boil.

4. Cover fish with 1/2 the butter mixture.

5. Sprinkle with lemon

pepper.

6. Cover with foil.

7. Bake 15 to 20 minutes in the preheated oven until fish is easily flaked with a fork.

8. Pour the remaining butter mixture over the fish to serve.

Baked Haddock in Cream Sauce

Prep time: 20 min | Cooking time: 40 min | Servings: 4

NUTRITION PER SERVING:

Calories 63 | Sodium 74mg | Protein 5.3g | Potassium 151mg | Phosphorus 116mg.

Ingredients

1 lb. haddock

½ cup all-purpose flour

2 tbsp. unsalted butter

¼ tsp. ground black pepper

2 cups fat-free nondairy creamer

¼ cup water.

Directions

1. Preheat your oven to 350°F. Spray baking pan with oil. Sprinkle with a little flour. Arrange fish on the pan.

2. Season with pepper. Sprinkle remaining flour on the fish. Spread creamer on both sides of the fish.

1. Bake for 40 minutes or until golden.

2. Spread cream sauce on top of the fish before serving.

Sweet Glazed Salmon

Prep time: 10 min | Cooking time: 10 min | Servings: 4

NUTRITION PER SERVING:

Calories: 240 | Fat: 15g | Sodium: 51mg | Carbs: 9g | Protein: 17 g | Potassium 265mg | Phosphorus 111mg.

Ingredients

2 tbsp. honey

1 tsp. lemon zest

½ tsp. ground black pepper

4 (3-ounce) salmon fillets

1 tbsp. olive oil

½, scallion, white and green parts, chopped.

Directions

1. In a bowl, stir together the lemon zest, honey, and pepper.

2. Wash the salmon and pat dry with paper towels. Rub the honey mixture all over each fillet.

3. In a large skillet, heat the olive oil. Add the salmon fillets and cook for 10 minutes, turning once, or until it is lightly browned and just cooked through.

4. Serve topped with chopped scallion.

Tilapia Fish Packets

Prep time: 15 min | Cooking time: 20 min | Servings: 3

NUTRITION PER SERVING:

Calories: 161 | Fat: 5.9g | Carbs: 6.4g | Protein: 22.3g | Sodium 216mg | Potassium 285mg | Phosphorus 54mg.

Ingredients

3 (4-ounce) tilapia fillets

½ tsp. cayenne pepper

½ tsp. salt

3 tsp. olive oil

1 red onion, sliced

3 lemon slices

1 zucchini, chopped.

Directions

1. Make the medium packets from the foil and brush them with olive oil from inside.

2. Then sprinkle tilapia fillets with salt and cayenne pepper from each side and arrange in the foil packets.

3. Add sliced lemon to the top of the fish.

4. Then add sliced onion and zucchini.

5. Bake the fish packets for 20 minutes at 360°F or until vegetables are tender.

Zesty Turkey

Prep time: 15 min | Cooking time: 30 min | Servings: 4

NUTRITION PER SERVING:

Calories 258 | Sodium 126mg | Protein 25.8g | Potassium 59mg | Phosphorus 50 mg.

Ingredients

¼ cup leek, chopped

2 tbsp. balsamic vinegar

2 tbsp. butter, melted

1 tsp. fresh oregano

½ tsp. garlic, minced

¼ tsp. ground black pepper

¼ tsp. paprika

8 oz. turkey breast, skinless and boneless.

Directions

6. Combine leek, herbs and seasonings.

7. Cut turkey breast into 2 pieces. Pour marinade over turkey in a plastic storage bag. Refrigerate and marinate from 30 minutes up to 24 hours.

8. Remove turkey from marinade. Pan Fry in medium-hot, non-stick, or greased skillet for several minutes on each side until thoroughly cooked. (Using a thermometer, the internal temperature of the turkey breast should be 170°F).

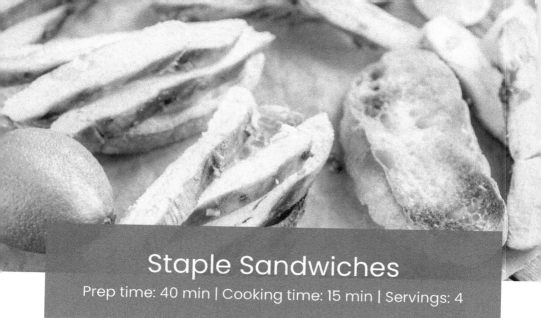

Staple Sandwiches

Prep time: 40 min | Cooking time: 15 min | Servings: 4

NUTRITION PER SERVING:

Calories: 239 | Fat: 8.5g | Carbs: 37.2g | Protein: 7g | Fiber: 5.6g | Potassium: 294mg | Sodium: 169mg.

Ingredients

3 tsp. low-sodium mayo

2 white bread slices, toasted

3 tbsp. unsalted turkey, cooked and chopped

2 thin apple slices

2 tbsp. low-fat Cheddar cheese

1 tsp. olive oil.

Directions

1. Spread mayonnaise over each slice evenly.

2. Place turkey over 1 slice, followed by apple slices and cheese.

3. Cover with the remaining slice to make a sandwich.

4. Grease a large nonstick frying pan with oil and heat on medium heat.

5. Place the sandwich in the

frying pan, and with the back of the spoon, gently press down.

6. Cook for about 1-2 minutes.

7. Carefully flip the whole sandwich and cook for about 1-2 minutes.

8. Transfer the sandwich to a serving plate.

9. With a knife, carefully cut the sandwich diagonally ad serve.

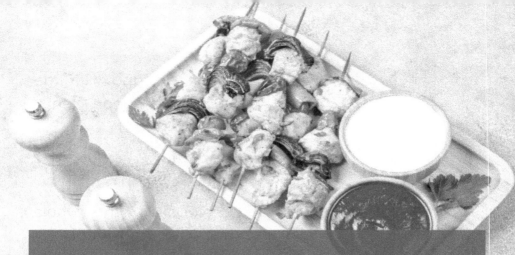

Chicken & Vegetables Kebabs

Prep time: 45 min | Cooking time: 15 min | Servings: 4

NUTRITION PER SERVING:

Calories: 284 | Fat: 16g | Carbs: 10g | Protein: 24g | Sodium: 215mg | Potassium: 456mg | Phosphorus 194mg.

Ingredients

2 tbsp. olive oil

1 tbsp. peach jam

2 tbsp. lemon juice

1 tsp. herb seasoning blend

¼ tsp. salt

1 lb. chicken thighs, boneless and skinless

1 zucchini

1 yellow summer

Directions

1. To make the marinade, microwave peach jam for 10 to 15 seconds to liquefy. Add the olive oil, lemon juice, herb seasoning and salt. Stir until well blended.

2. Rinse the chicken thighs and pat dry with a paper towel. Cut each thigh into 4 pieces and place in bowl. Add 3 tablespoons marinade to the chicken

squash

1 medium onion

1 red bell pepper.

pieces. Cover and refrigerate for 30 minutes to marinate.

3. Cut the vegetables into even bite-sized pieces for the kebabs (zucchini-8 slices; squash-8 slices; pepper-16 pieces; onion-varies). Place them in a bowl and add 2 tablespoons marinade. Stir to coat the vegetable pieces.

4. Thread the vegetables and chicken pieces onto skewers (4 large or 8 small skewers).

5. Heat the grill to medium heat. Place the skewers on the grill and cook covered for 12 to 15 minutes. Turn the skewers 2 or 3 times to cook evenly.

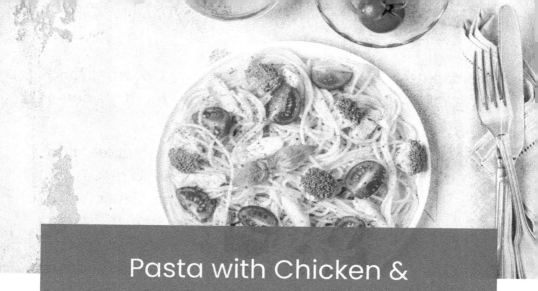

Pasta with Chicken & Vegetables

Prep time: 30 min | Cooking time: 25 min | Servings: 2

NUTRITION PER SERVING:

Calories 250 | Protein 15g | Carbs 28g | Fiber 3.7g | Fat 9g | Cholesterol 22mg | Sodium 265mg | Potassium 329mg | Phosphorus 140 mg.

Ingredients

1 tbsp. olive oil

½ cup green bell pepper

¼ cup onion

½ tsp. garlic powder

½ cup fresh broccoli florets

1 tsp. dried

Directions

1. Chop bell pepper and onion.

2. Dice chicken.

3. Place oil in a large nonstick frying pan and stir-fry the bell pepper, onion and broccoli.

4. Sprinkle with the

rosemary

1 tbsp. fresh basil

¼ tsp. red pepper flakes

⅛ tsp. salt

2 oz. chicken, cooked

¼ cup low-sodium chicken broth

2 tsp. cornstarch

1 cup pasta twists, cooked.

rosemary, basil, red pepper flakes, garlic powder and salt.

5. Stir in the cooked chicken.

6. Mix chicken broth with cornstarch and add to vegetable and chicken mixture. Cook until thickened slightly.

7. Stir in the cup of hot cooked pasta.

8. Remove from heat and serve.

Notes: For quick preparation, use 1¼ cups of a frozen vegetable mixture of similar composition to replace fresh vegetables.

Squeeze on lemon juice or sprinkle with balsamic vinegar to add a tangy flavor.

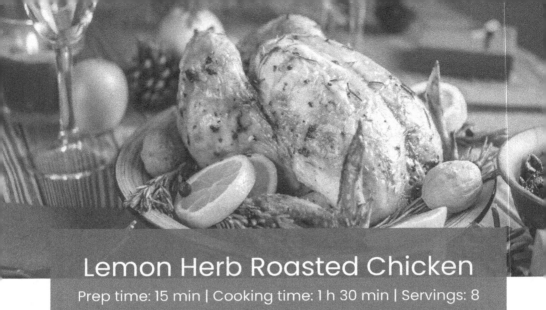

Lemon Herb Roasted Chicken

Prep time: 15 min | Cooking time: 1 h 30 min | Servings: 8

NUTRITION PER SERVING:

Calories 188 | Fat 9g | Carbs 20g | Fiber 6g | Protein 45g | Sodium 178mg | Potassium 376mg | Phosphorus 266 mg.

Ingredients

- ½ tsp. ground black pepper
- ½ tsp. mustard powder
- ½ tsp. salt
- 1 (3-lb) whole chicken
- 1 tsp. garlic powder
- 2 lemons
- 2 tbsp. olive oil

Directions

1. Preheat your oven to 350°F.

2. In a small bowl, mix well black pepper, garlic powder, mustard powder, and salt.

3. Rinse chicken well and slice off giblets. In a greased 9x13-inches baking dish, place chicken and add 1½ tablespoon of seasoning

2 tsp. Italian seasoning.

made earlier inside the chicken and rub the remaining seasoning around the chicken.

4. In a small bowl, mix olive oil and juice from 2 lemons. Drizzle over chicken.

5. Bake chicken until juices run clear, around 1 hour 30 minutes.

6. Every once in a while, baste the chicken with its juices.

7. Serve hot.

Chicken Marsala

Prep time: 10 min | Cooking time: 15 min | Servings: 4

NUTRITION PER SERVING:

Calories 121 | Sodium 76mg | Protein 1.9g | Potassium 162mg | Phosphorus 115mg.

Ingredients

4 chicken breast fillets

½ cup all-purpose flour

2 tbsp. olive oil

½ cup shallots, chopped

2 cups fresh mushrooms, sliced

5 tbsp. fresh parsley, chopped

1 tbsp. butter mixed with 1 tbsp. olive oil

¼ cup dry Marsala wine

¼ tsp. garlic powder

⅛ tsp. black pepper.

Directions

1. Coat both sides of chicken with flour.

2. Cook in hot oil in a pan over medium heat, until golden or for 5 minutes per side.

3. Put the chicken on a platter and set aside.

4. Sauté mushrooms, parsley, and shallots in olive oil butter blend for 3 minutes.

5. Add the rest of the ingredients. Simmer for 2 minutes.

6. Pour sauce over chicken and serve with white rice.

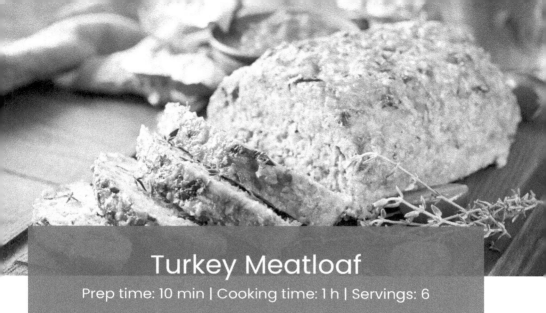

Turkey Meatloaf

Prep time: 10 min | Cooking time: 1 h | Servings: 6

NUTRITION PER SERVING:

Calories 197 | Sodium 305mg | Protein 20g | Carbs 9g | Fat 9g |
Potassium 314mg | Phosphorus 206mg.

Ingredients

1 lb. ground turkey,
7% fat

3 oz. turkey
sausage

1 whole egg + 1
egg white

½ cup dry
breadcrumbs

¼ cup fresh
parsley, chopped

1 tbsp.

Directions

1. Preheat oven to 350°F.

2. Combine all ingredients in a large bowl and mix well.

3. Transfer to a greased 9x5-inches loaf pan and bake for 1 hour.

4. Slice into 6 equal pieces and serve.

Worcestershire sauce

1 tsp. Italian seasoning

½ tsp. black pepper.

Goulash

Prep time: 30 min | Cooking time: 30 min | Servings: 6

NUTRITION PER SERVING:

Calories: 471 | Fat: 17g | Carbs: 53g | Protein: 20g | Potassium: 462mg | Sodium: 43mg | Phosphorus 216mg.

Ingredients

8 oz. pork loin, cubed

¼ cup olive oil

1 cup onion, chopped

3 garlic cloves, minced

2 tbsp. unbleached flour

2 tsp. paprika

1 cup dry white wine

1 tbsp. tomato paste

1 cup green pepper, sliced

1 cup mushrooms,

Directions

1. In a medium skillet, brown the meat in the olive oil over medium heat.

2. Add the onions and garlic.

1. Stir in flour and paprika.

2. Whisk in the wine and tomato paste and incorporate well.

3. Add in the peppers, mushrooms, carrots and water. Simmer until pork is tender, about 10-15 minutes.

4. Season with pepper and salt, if desired.

5. While the goulash is cooking, cook the noodles

sliced

2 small carrots, sliced

3-4 cups water

Ground black paper, to taste

12 oz. egg noodles (6 cups of cooked pasta)

½ tbsp. butter.

in a separate pot until al dente. Drain and add the butter to moisten and keep the noodles from sticking. Cover and set aside.

6. Serve the cooked stew over the noodles and enjoy!

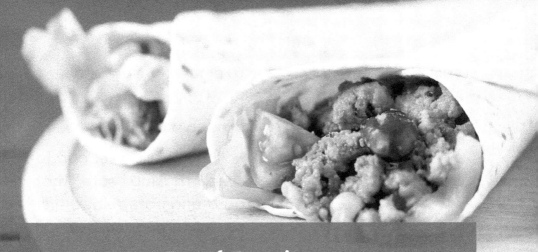

Beef Burritos

Prep time: 10 min | Cooking time: 20 min | Servings: 6

NUTRITION PER SERVING:

Calories 265 | Sodium 341mg | Protein 15g | Carbs 31g | Fat 9g | Potassium 303mg | Phosphorus 172mg.

Ingredients

¼ cup onion, chopped

¼ cup green pepper, chopped

1 lb. lean ground beef

¼ cup low-sodium tomato puree

¼ tsp. ground black pepper

¼ tsp. ground

Directions

1. In a medium skillet, brown ground beef; drain on paper towels.

2. Spray skillet with non-stick cooking spray; add onion and green pepper and cook for 3 to 5 minutes, until vegetables are softened.

3. Add beef, tomato puree, black pepper and cumin. Mix well and cook for 3 to

cumin

6 burrito size flour tortillas.

5 minutes on low heat.

4. Divide the beef mixture among 6 tortillas.

5. Roll the tortilla over burrito style, making sure that both ends are folded first so mixture does not fall out.

Stuffed Peppers

Prep time: 20 min | Cooking time: 1 h | Servings: 8

NUTRITION PER SERVING:

Calories 208 | Protein 17g | Carbs 17g | Fat 8g | Sodium 109mg | Potassium 615mg | Phosphorus 143mg.

Ingredients

8 bell peppers

1 lb. ground beef

1 onion, finely chopped

1 cup leftover rice

1 can tomato paste

1 tsp. oregano dried

1 tbsp. parsley, chopped.

Directions

1. Preheat oven to 350°F.

2. Cut off tops of peppers and scoop out seeds and pith.

3. Mix beef, onion, rice, tomato paste, and herbs together.

4. Fill peppers and put tops back on.

5. Pour 1/2 cup water in bottom of casserole dish and add the peppers.

6. Bake about 1 hour.

Mediterranean Meatballs

Prep time: 15 min | Cooking time: 35 min | Servings: 4

NUTRITION PER SERVING:

Calories 161 | Sodium 145mg | Protein 21g | Carbs 3g | Fat 6g | Potassium 321mg | Phosphorus 213mg.

Ingredients

Olive oil cooking spray

12 oz. lean ground beef

1 egg

2 tbsp. breadcrumbs

2 tbsp. Parmesan, grated

1 tbsp. fresh parsley, chopped

1 tsp. garlic, minced

½ tsp. Dijon mustard

Pinch of black pepper.

Directions

1. Preheat the oven to 350°F. Lightly coat a baking sheet with cooking spray.

2. In a large bowl, mix together the beef, breadcrumbs, egg, Parmesan cheese, parsley, garlic, mustard, and pepper.

3. Form the meat mixture into small (1-inch) meatballs and arrange them on the prepared baking sheet.

4. Bake until browned, turning several times, about 35 minutes. Serve hot.

Kidney Friendly Lasagna

Prep time: 20 min | Cooking time: 40 min | Servings: 8

NUTRITION PER SERVING:

Calories: 487 | Fat: 2.9g | Carbs: 44g | Protein: 24.9g | Fiber: 2.7g | Potassium: 491mg | Phosphorus 242mg | Sodium: 214mg.

Ingredients

1 lb. lean ground beef

8 oz. whipped cream cheese, softened

½ cup Parmesan cheese, grated

2 large eggs

1 small Roma tomato, diced

½ cup Portabella mushroom, sliced

½ cup zucchini, sliced

½ cup kale, chopped

1 tsp. garlic, crushed

Directions

5. Preheat oven 375° F.

6. Brown ground beef in a skillet.

7. In a medium bowl combine cooked ground beef, 1 egg, 1/4 cup water, garlic, basil and oregano. Mix with 3 tablespoons olive oil.

8. In another bowl, combine softened cream cheese, Parmesan cheese, 1 egg and 1/2-cup water. Mix well.

9. Sauté mushrooms and kale in remaining tablespoon olive oil.

1 tbsp. dried basil

1 tbsp. dried oregano

4 tbsp. olive oil

8 oven ready lasagna noodles.

10. In an 11x7-inches pan, spread 1/4 of the ground beef mixture on bottom of pan.

11. Top with 4 uncooked lasagna noodles.

12. Spread half the cream cheese mixture, about 1/4-inch thick, over noodles.

13. Layer zucchini, sautéed mushrooms, kale and remaining ground beef mixture evenly over noodles.

14. Repeat noodle and cream cheese layer.

15. Top with diced tomato. Cover with foil and bake for 30 minutes.

16. Remove foil and bake for additional 10-15 minutes.

17. Let stand for 10 minutes, cut into 8 portions and serve.

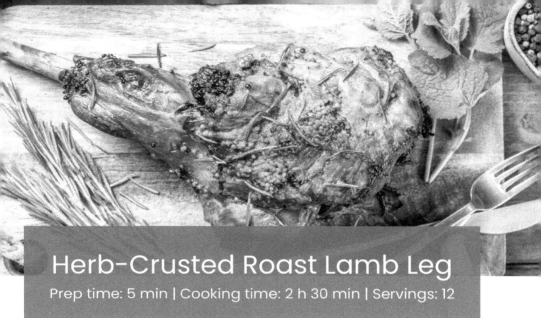

Herb-Crusted Roast Lamb Leg

Prep time: 5 min | Cooking time: 2 h 30 min | Servings: 12

NUTRITION PER SERVING:

Calories 292 | Protein 24g | Carbs 2g | Fat 20g | Sodium 157mg | Potassium 419mg | Phosphorus 232mg.

Ingredients

1 (4-pound) lamb leg

3 tbsp. lemon juice

1 tbsp. curry powder

2 garlic cloves, minced

½ tsp. ground black pepper

1 cup onions, sliced

Directions

1. Preheat oven to 400° F.
2. Place leg of lamb on a roasting pan. Sprinkle with 1 teaspoon of lemon juice.
3. Make paste with 2 teaspoons of lemon juice and the rest of the spices.
4. Rub the paste onto the lamb.
5. Roast lamb for 30 minutes.

½ *cup dry vermouth.*

6. Drain off fat and add vermouth and onions. Reduce heat to 325°F and cook for an additional 1¾–2 hours.

7. Baste leg of lamb frequently. When internal temperature is 145°F, remove from oven and let rest 3 minutes before serving.

Roast Pork Loin & Apple Stuffing

Prep time: 20 min | Cooking time: 1 h| Servings: 6

NUTRITION PER SERVING:

Calories: 263 | Fat: 14g | Carbs: 22g | Protein: 14g | Potassium: 275mg | Phosphorus 154mg | Sodium: 137mg.

Ingredients

FOR APPLE
STUFFING:

2 tbsp. canola oil

2 cups packed cubed white bread

½ cup finely diced Granny Smith apple

2 tbsp. unsalted butter

2 tbsp. onions, finely diced

2 tbsp. celery, finely diced

½ tsp. dried thyme

1 tsp. ground black pepper

½ cup low-sodium

Directions

ROAST PORK LOIN:

1. Preheat oven to 400°F.

1. Sauté all ingredients in canola oil except for chicken stock for 2–3 minutes in large sauté pan on medium-high heat.

2. Slowly add chicken broth until moist, but not too wet. (You may not need it all, depending on how much juice is released from the apples during cooking.) Remove from heat and chill to room temperature.

3. Meanwhile, cut 5 slits

chicken broth.

<u>FOR ROAST PORK LOIN:</u>

1 lb. pork loin, boneless

2 (18-inch) pieces of butcher twine.

<u>FOR CHERRY MARMALADE GLAZE:</u>

½ cup sugar-free orange marmalade

¼ cup apple juice

¼ cup dried cherries

⅛ tsp. cinnamon

⅛ tsp. nutmeg.

about 1 inch apart along the length of the loin, forming several pockets.

4. Stuff each pocket with about 2 tablespoons of stuffing (there should be a little left over).

5. Tie 1 long piece of twine around the length of the loin and tie additional twine across the shorter length as needed to keep the stuffing in place.

6. Place remaining stuffing on a baking sheet tray, place tied stuffed pork on top and bake for 45 minutes at 400°F or until you reach an internal temperature of 160°F.

7. Spoon on the dried cherry marmalade glaze, shut oven heat off and let rest in oven for 10–15 minutes. Remove pork loin, slice into portions then serve.

<u>CHERRY MARMALADE GLAZE:</u>

8. Mix all the glaze

ingredients in a small saucepan on medium-high heat until marmalade is melted and starts to simmer. Turn off heat and set aside.

DESSERT
RECIPES

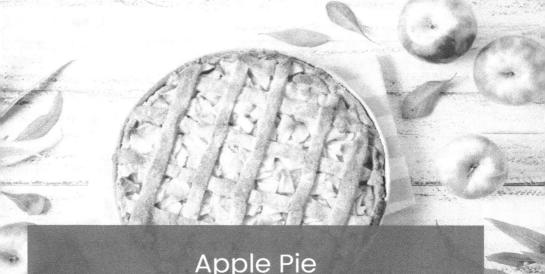

Apple Pie

Prep time: 10 min | Cooking time: 50 min | Servings: 6

NUTRITION PER SERVING:

Calories 517 | Protein 4g | Carbohydrates 51g | Fat 33g | Cholesterol 24mg | Sodium 65mg | Potassium 145mg | Phosphorus 43mg | Calcium 24mg | Fiber 2.7g.

Ingredients

6 medium apples, peeled, cored and sliced

½ cup granulated sugar

1 tsp. ground cinnamon

6 tbsp. unsalted butter

2⅔ cups all-

Directions

1. Preheat your oven to 425°F.

2. Toss the apple slices with cinnamon and sugar in a bowl and set it aside covered.

3. Blend the flour with the shortening in a pastry blender, then add chilled water by the tablespoon.

*purpose white
flour*

1 cup shortening

6 tbsp. water.

4. Continue mixing and adding the water until it forms a smooth dough ball.

5. Divide the dough into 2 equal-size pieces and spread them into 2 separate 9-inch sheets.

6. Arrange the sheet of dough at the bottom of a 9-inch pie pan.

7. Spread the apples in the pie shell and spread a tablespoon of butter over it.

8. Cover the filling with the remaining sheet of the dough and pinch down the edges.

9. Carve 1-inch cuts on top of the pie.

10. Bake for 50 minutes or until golden.

11. Slice and serve.

Cashew Cheese Bites

Prep time: 5 min | Cooking time: 5 min | Servings: 12

NUTRITION PER SERVING:

Calories 192 | Fat 17.1g | Carbs 6.5g | Protein 5.2g | Sodium: 10mg | Potassium 93mg | Phosphorus 37mg.

Ingredients

8 oz. cream cheese

1 tsp. cinnamon

1 cup cashew butter.

Directions

1. Add all ingredients into the blender and blend until smooth.

2. Pour blended mixture into the mini muffin liners and place them in the refrigerator until set.

3. Serve and enjoy.

Banana Pudding Dessert

Prep time: 1 h 10 min | Cooking time: 5 min | Servings: 4

NUTRITION PER SERVING:

Calories 270 | Protein 2g | Carbs 54g | Fat 5g | Sodium 50mg | Potassium 85mg | Phosphorus 26mg.

Ingredients

12 oz. vanilla wafers

2 boxes banana cream pudding mix

2½ cups unenriched rice milk

8 oz. dairy whipped topping.

Directions

1. Line the bottom of a 9x13-inch pan with a layer of wafers.

2. Mix the banana pudding mix with 2.5 cups of milk in a saucepan. Bring it to a boil while constantly stirring. Pour over the wafers.

3. Add another layer of wafers over the pudding layer and press them down gently. Place the layered pudding in the refrigerator for 1 hour.

4. Garnish with whipped cream and serve.

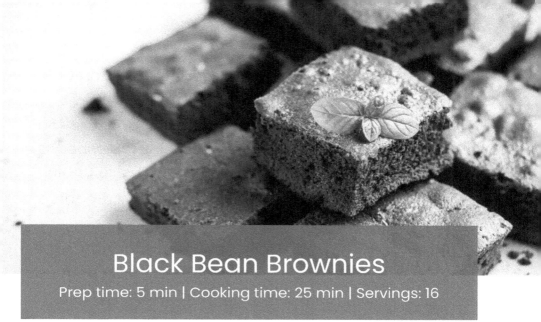

Black Bean Brownies

Prep time: 5 min | Cooking time: 25 min | Servings: 16

NUTRITION PER SERVING:

Calories 113 | Protein 3g | Carbs 18g | Fiber: 4.6 g | Fat 4.7g | Sodium 191mg | Potassium 176mg | Phosphorus 142mg.

Ingredients

Vegetable cooking spray

2 large eggs, beaten

1 (15-oz.) can black beans, rinsed and drained

3 tbsp. vegetable oil

¾ cup cocoa

Directions

1. Preheat your oven to 350°F. Spray an 8x8-inch baking dish with vegetable oil cooking spray.

2. In a food processor combine all the ingredients (besides toppings) and puree for about 3 minutes, scraping down sides and

powder

¼ tsp. salt

1 tsp. pure vanilla extract

¼ tsp. stevia

1½ tsp. low-sodium baking powder.

TOPPINGS (optional)

Crushed walnuts

Pecans

Chocolate chips.

processing to a creamy batter.

3. If the batter appears too thick, add 1-2 tablespoons of water and pulse again.

4. Pour batter into prepared pan.

5. Optional: Sprinkle with crushed walnuts, pecans or chocolate chips.

6. Bake until toothpick inserted 2 inches from center tests done, 18 to 25 minutes.

7. Cool completely before cutting into 16 (2-inch) squares.

Spiced Peaches

Prep time: 5 min | Cooking time: 10 min | Servings: 2

NUTRITION PER SERVING:

Calories: 70 | Carbs 14g | Phosphorus 23mg | Potassium: 176mg | Sodium: 3mg | Protein: 1g.

Ingredients

1 cup canned peaches with juices

½ tsp. cornstarch

1 tsp. ground cloves

1 tsp. ground cinnamon

1 tsp. ground nutmeg

½ lemon zest

½ cup water.

Directions

1. Drain peaches.

1. Combine cinnamon, cornstarch, nutmeg, ground cloves, and lemon zest in a pan on the stove.

2. Heat on medium heat and add peaches.

3. Bring to a boil, reduce the heat and simmer for 10 minutes.

4. Serve.

No-Bake Protein Balls

Prep time: 5 min | Cooking time: 5 min | Servings: 12

NUTRITION PER SERVING:

Calories 179 | Fat 14.8g | Carbohydrates 10.1g | Protein 7g | Sodium 69mg | Potassium 214mg.

Ingredients

¾ cup peanut butter

1 tsp. cinnamon

3 tbsp. erythritol

1½ cup almond flour.

Directions

1. Add all ingredients into the mixing bowl and blend until well combined.

2. Place bowl into the fridge for 30 minutes.

3. Remove bowl from the fridge. Make small balls from the mixture and place on a baking dish.

4. Serve and enjoy.

CPSIA information can be obtained
at www.ICGtesting.com
Printed in the USA
BVHW071804230621
610293BV00014B/2238